TEEN LIFE™

FREQUENTLY ASKED QUESTIONS ABOUT

Celiac Disease

Terry L. Smith

ROSEN PUBLISHING®
New York

Published in 2007 by The Rosen Publishing Group, Inc.
29 East 21st Street, New York, NY 10010

First Edition

Library of Congress Cataloging-in-Publication Data

Smith, Terry L. (Terry Lane), 1944–
Frequently asked questions about celiac disease / Terry L. Smith. — 1st ed.
p. cm. — (FAQ—teen life)
Includes bibliographical references and index.
ISBN-13: 978-1-4042-0962-6
ISBN-10: 1-4042-0962-X (library binding)
1. Celiac disease–Popular works. I. Title.
RC862.C44S65 2007
616.3'99—dc22

2006021358

Manufactured in the United States of America

Contents

Introduction

Imagine turning on your TV and hearing the announcer excitedly report that a panic is overtaking the country. Thousands upon thousands of people have just learned they have a mysterious disease. Doctors' offices and hospital emergency rooms are swamped, as these new patients try to find out what's wrong with them. The Internet is shut down due to an overload of queries seeking information on a strange new word, "gluten." Grocery stores across the country report they're not able to keep bananas, rice, and corn chips on the shelves due to increased demand. The president of the United States has made an appeal for calm, pointing out that, while this disease has no cure, it is quite treatable. People only have to be careful about what they eat. Leading medical experts have fanned out to speak at public gatherings, reassuring patients that their medical condition is not some exotic new disease. Doctors have known a great deal about it and how to treat it for years. They just didn't know that so many people were affected by it.

Is this an unlikely scenario? Sure it is. But it's interesting to think what would happen if everyone who has celiac disease suddenly discovered that they have it. Scientists estimate that as many as 1 out of every 100 to 150 people may have celiac disease, but only about 3 percent of those cases have been diagnosed. It is a serious, lifelong disease that affects

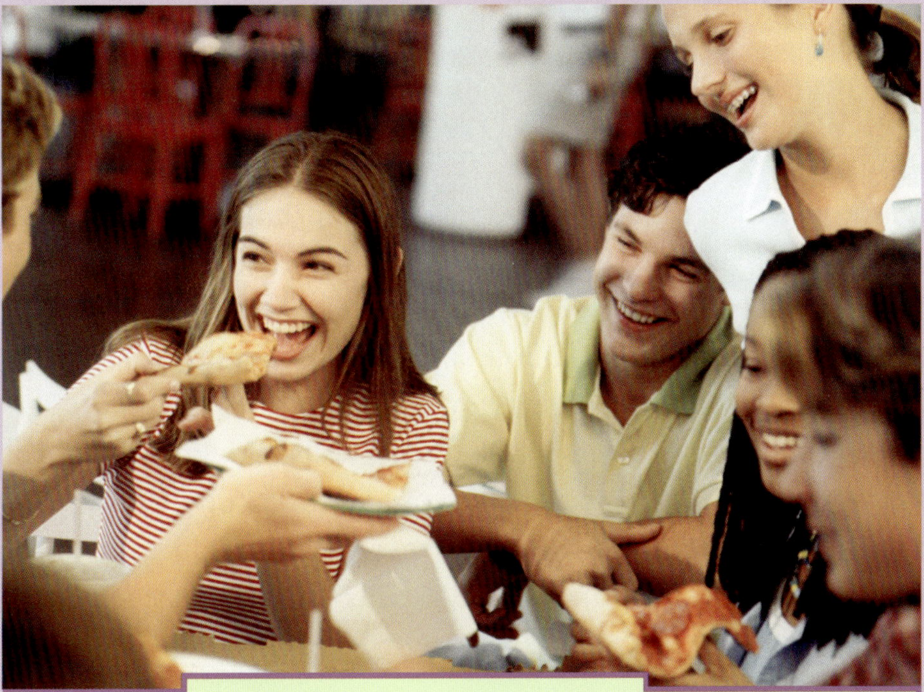

Many happy occasions involve sharing a meal, such as these teenagers enjoying a pizza party. If you have celiac disease, you know how to plan ahead so you can enjoy the fun and keep to a healthy diet.

the body's ability to process certain foods (those with gluten). It causes a wide range of symptoms, many of which are associated with the intestinal system, like diarrhea, bloating, and weight loss. Celiac disease often occurs in young children, but it may be diagnosed in adolescence and throughout adulthood.

Many people have the disease and don't know it. This is because the symptoms are confusable with many other diseases. For some people, there are no symptoms at all. Also, most doctors still think of it as a rare disease and may not even test for it.

The treatment for celiac disease, once it is diagnosed, is straightforward and always the same, no matter a person's age or symptoms. The treatment is to eat a diet that doesn't contain gluten. Gluten is a protein found in wheat, rye, and barley. When a person has celiac disease, gluten acts like a poison inside the intestines. If the person eats a diet that is totally gluten-free, the affected tissues in the small intestine heal, and symptoms of the disease disappear rapidly. Generally, if you meet a person with celiac disease, you would never know she has it, except that you may notice she is careful to eat a diet that's healthy for her. Other than that, she leads a totally normal life.

Chapter one

WHAT IS CELIAC DISEASE?

Celiac disease, also referred to as coeliac disease or nontropical sprue, is a genetic autoimmune disease that affects the digestive system and its ability to obtain nutrients from food. The name "celiac" comes from a Greek word having to do with the abdominal cavity. The function of the digestive system is disrupted if a common food ingredient, called gluten, reaches the small intestine. When this happens, the body's immune system gets a signal that tells it to begin attacking the intestinal lining, eventually destroying the cells that enable the body to take nutrients from food.

Normal Digestive Process

The digestive system can be thought of in its simplest form as a long tube coiled inside the body, with food

This diagram shows the principal parts of the digestive system. Celiac disease affects the upper portion of the small intestine.

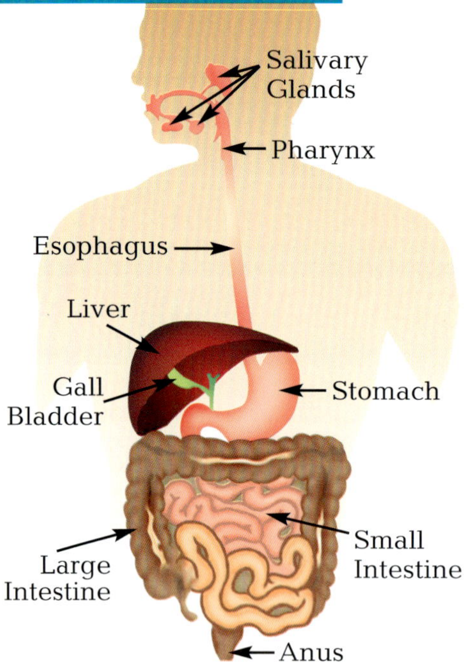

entering at one end, the mouth, and waste products exiting at the other end, the anus. In reality, it is a complex system on which our bodies depend for all essential nutrients. The system is able to process the huge variety of foods we take in, extracting from it the nutrients the body requires, then eliminating the rest. Our food consists of six types of nutrients: protein, carbohydrates, fat, vitamins, minerals, and water. It is important that we eat the proper amount of each of these—in other words, a balanced diet. Our intestines must be able to absorb each of these elements and pass them to the parts of the body that require them.

The digestive process begins in the mouth with the production of saliva by the salivary glands. The saliva helps to hold chewed food together as it passes through the pharynx and esophagus to the stomach. It also contains enzymes that start the process of digesting, or breaking down, food. Once we have chewed and swallowed our food, involuntary muscles take over to slowly move the food through the length of the gastrointestinal tract. The action of these muscles is referred to as peristalsis.

As we eat, the stomach receives a signal to begin producing gastric acid. It will continue the digestive process as soon as the chewed food reaches it. Gastric acid also kills bacteria and inactivates toxins that may have been in our food.

Food passes from the stomach to the first part of the small intestine, which is the duodenum. It is here that the essential function of absorbing nutrients from our food begins. The arrival of food stimulates the production of enzymes and fluids that chemically convert the contents of our food to forms that can be absorbed into the bloodstream. These chemical processes are at work as peristalsis slowly moves food through the length of the small intestine. At the same time, the cells lining the small intestine are taking up, or absorbing, the chemicals produced by the enzymatic action. In order for there to be enough cells to absorb all the nutrients needed by the body, the inside of the small intestine is lined with millions of tiny fingerlike projections called villi. The surfaces of these villi are covered by epithelial cells that take in chemical nutrients. These cells are produced in the crypts, or "valleys," between the villi. The villi greatly increase the surface area of the small intestine, which increases the body's capacity for nutrient intake. Inside the villi are blood and lymph vessels. In normal digestion, chemical nutrients are transported through the epithelial cells, into the vessels, and then to the rest of the body. If any bacteria or toxic substances are taken into the villi, white blood cells and chemical messengers

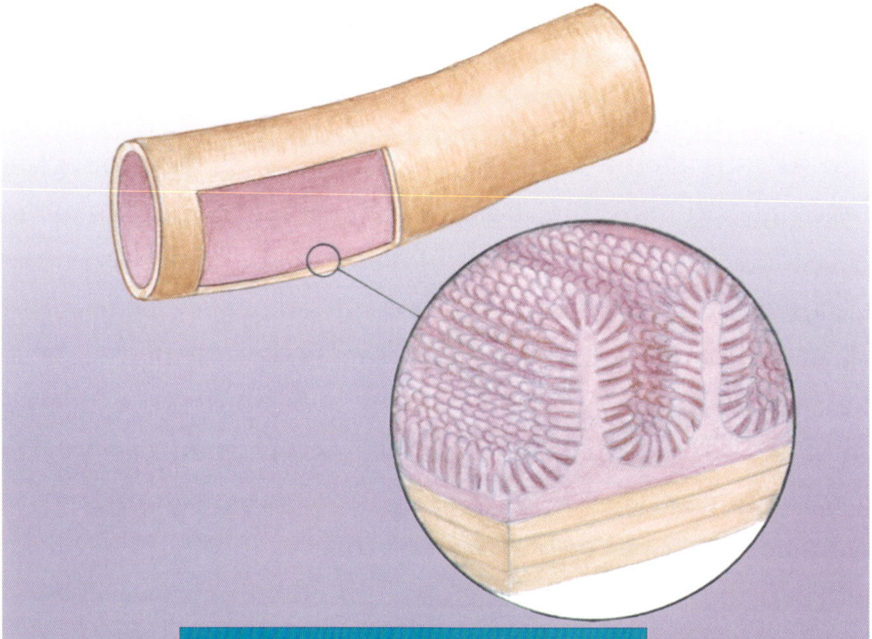

The lining of the small intestine has millions of tiny projections called villi, shown in this drawing. The villi play an important role in the absorption of nutrients.

notify the body's immune system to mount an attack against these invaders.

By the time digested food passes through the jejunum (middle part of the small intestine) and the ileum (final part of the small intestine), most of the nutrients have been absorbed. Each part of the small intestine plays a special role in absorbing certain nutrients. For example, protein and calcium (among other things) are absorbed in the duodenum and jejunum. Since most foods contain a portion of non-digestible matter, there are some contents remaining after passage through the small intestine.

This non-digested material, called fecal matter, passes to the colon, or large intestine, in preparation for being eliminated. During transit through the colon, water is absorbed from the fecal matter, leaving only the solid contents we know as stools or bowel movements. This material is stored in the final section of the colon, known as the rectum, prior to discharge through the anus.

With such a complex process, it's no wonder that things sometimes go wrong. Usually, it's a matter of getting a stomachache from eating too much, or catching the flu from someone. After a few days, the system gets back to normal. But having celiac disease is quite a different matter, and it doesn't go away.

What Goes Wrong in Celiac Disease?

How can something as simple as a slice of bread cause so much trouble? Gluten is a general term for the protein part of wheat, rye, and barley. All proteins are made up of long chains of amino acids that must be broken down into smaller pieces by the enzymes of the gastrointestinal tract. The amino acid chain of gluten that causes the problem in celiac disease goes by the chemical name of gliadin. In the normal digestive process, amino acids are absorbed by the cells lining the villi of the small intestine, and are transported to wherever they are needed in the body. For a person with celiac disease, the gliadin is not broken down, but is converted by a particular enzyme called tissue transglutaminase (TTG) into a more toxic form. TTG is a key substance that enables physicians to make a diagnosis of celiac disease, as we will learn in chapter 2.

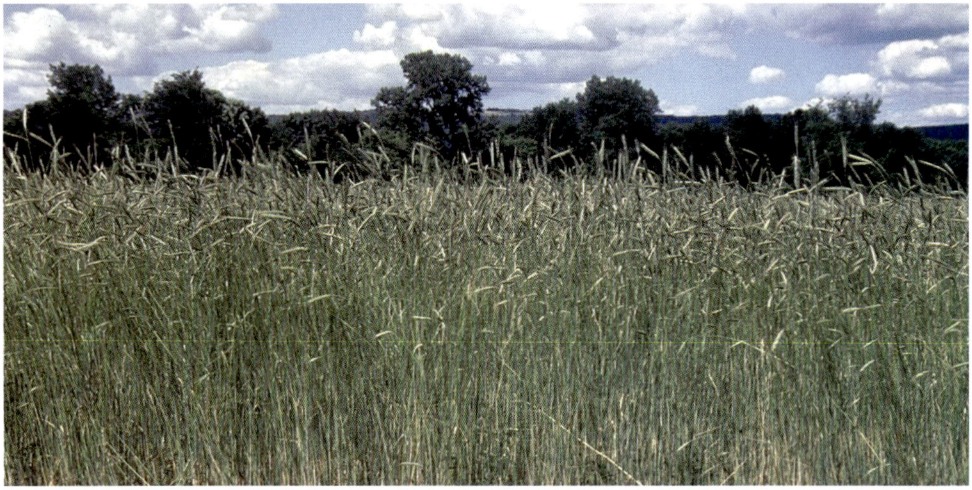

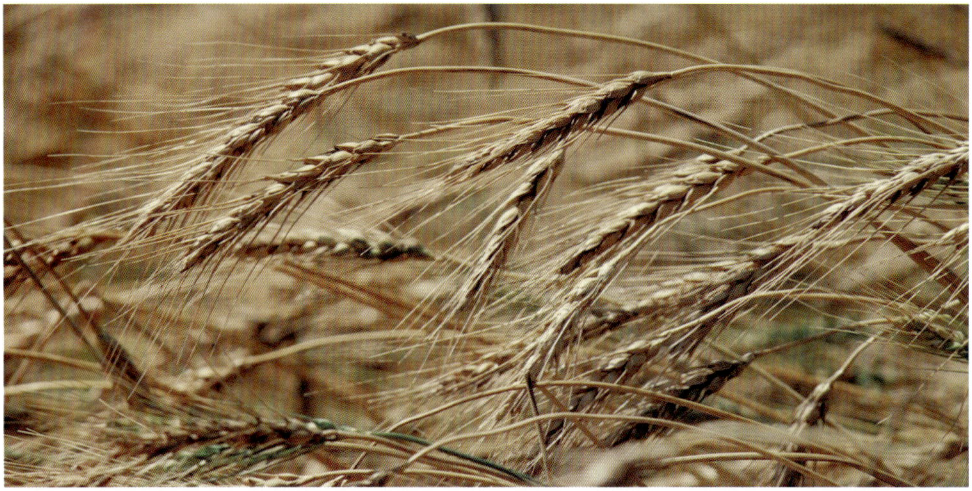

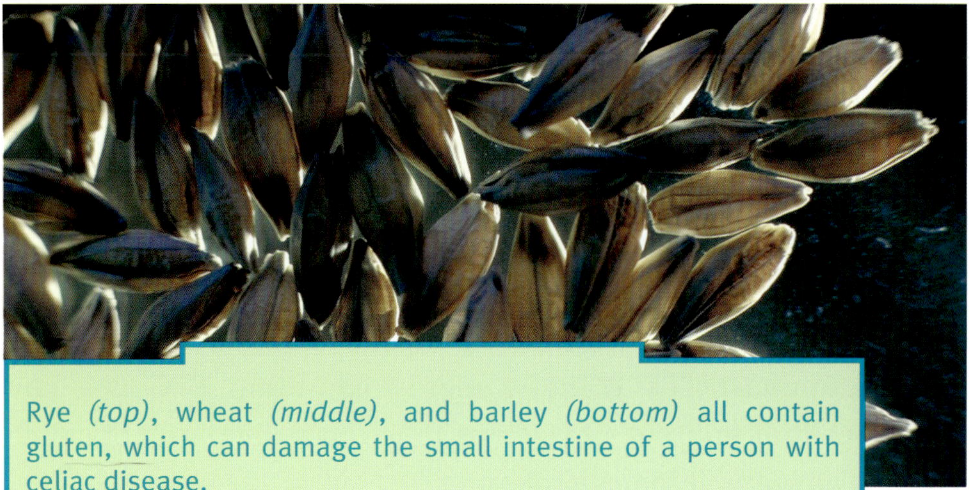

Rye *(top)*, wheat *(middle)*, and barley *(bottom)* all contain gluten, which can damage the small intestine of a person with celiac disease.

This toxic form of gliadin is able to make its way between the cells lining the villi. The white blood cells inside the villi recognize the gliadin as a toxic substance. They signal the immune system that an inflammatory reaction is required to repel the invader. If such an inflammatory process lasts only a short while, as when a person eats some bad food, the digestive system quickly returns to normal. But when a person has celiac disease and continues to eat food that contains gluten, the inflammatory process becomes so severe that the villi begin to shrink, or flatten. Over a period of months and years, so many villi are damaged in this way that the body can no longer absorb all the nutrients it requires from food passing through the gastrointestinal tract. A disease that acts in this way, causing the body's immune system to attack its own body cells, is called an autoimmune disease. This is different from an allergic reaction, in which the body mounts an immediate, short-term response to a substance to which it is allergic.

A Genetic Disease

Scientists have learned that everyone with celiac disease has certain abnormalities in their genetic makeup. All the cells of our body contain thousands of genes that are inherited from our parents. These genes control cell activities. The two known genetic features shared by persons with celiac disease have been labeled "HLA-DQ2" and "HLA-DQ8" by scientists. Still, about 30 percent of people have these genetic features and many never develop celiac disease. Why? We don't know the

10 FACTS ABOUT CELIAC DISEASE

1. Thousands of people have celiac disease and don't know it.
2. Celiac disease is life-long, with no known cure.
3. Celiac disease can be diagnosed at any age.
4. As many as 1 in 100 people may have celiac disease.
5. The only treatment for celiac disease is a gluten-free diet.
6. Gluten is a hidden ingredient in many processed foods.
7. Gluten can cause damage to the body, even when there are no symptoms.
8. One form of celiac disease causes an itchy rash.

9 Celiac disease is not a wheat allergy.

10 Persons with celiac disease learn there's a lot more to life than just eating.

answer yet. Scientists have learned that, in addition to genetics, a triggering event must occur for an individual to develop the disease. Researchers are trying to find out just what these triggers might be. If we could prevent the triggers in those who have a genetic predisposition for celiac disease, it would keep these persons from developing the disease. So far, evidence suggests that certain early-childhood events can influence whether a person with a genetic predisposition develops celiac disease. Breast-feeding of babies may have some protective effect. The amount of gluten and when it is first added to a baby's diet may also play a role. Damage to the lining of the intestine by an infection may bring on celiac disease. Pregnancy and other stressful effects on the body may also be related.

A Possible Cure?

Studies show that many people with celiac disease continue to eat gluten, either by choice or unknowingly. If you have celiac disease, you know what a relief it would be to eat without having

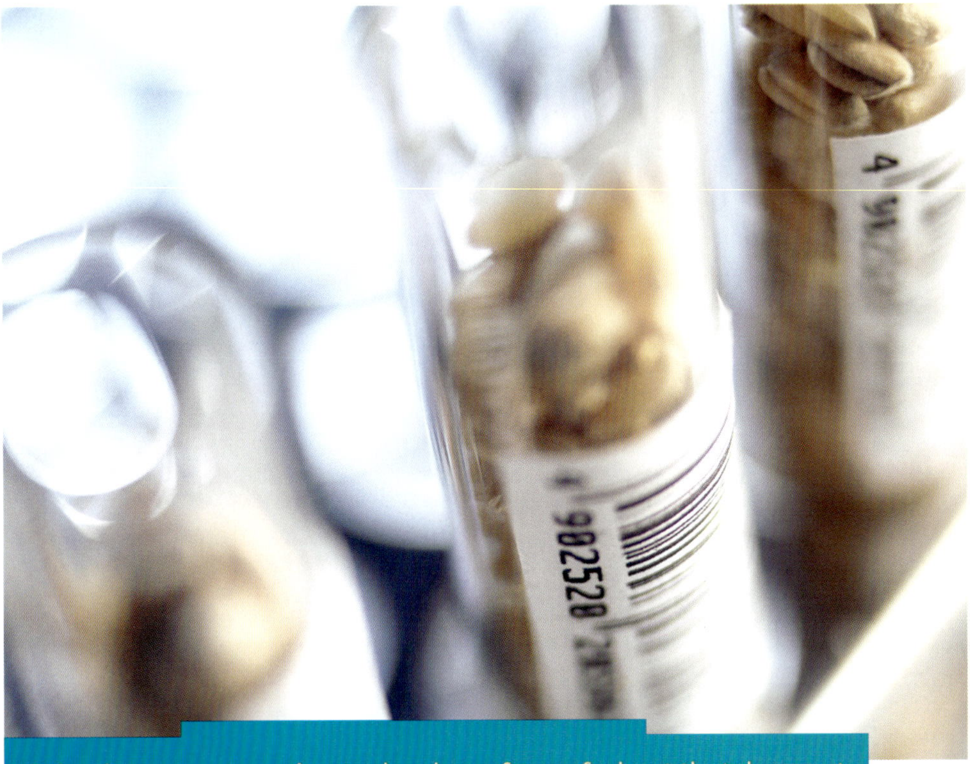

Scientists are attempting to develop a form of wheat that does not contain gluten. This photo shows wheat grains under study in a laboratory.

to think about gluten at every meal. Now that researchers understand more about gluten, it may be possible to interrupt the digestive process to weaken or destroy gluten's bad effects. One solution scientists are working on is the genetic alteration of wheat so that it no longer contains gluten. Other possibilities are medicines that could break down gliadin (the toxic portion of gluten) in the intestine, or interfere with the immune response to gliadin. Also in the works is a vaccine that blocks the immune response to gluten. Progress is being made, but it may be years before any of these options are available. Fortunately, current treatment of celiac disease (that is, being gluten-free) is very effective.

chapter two

DO I HAVE CELIAC DISEASE?

Just about everyone occasionally has some of the symptoms associated with celiac disease. The classic case of the disease involves the gastrointestinal tract, usually with stomachache, diarrhea, or cramps, and bloating of the intestines. If you don't have celiac disease, you can usually count on a stomachache or diarrhea going away in a day or two—as soon as a stray "bug" works its way out of the system. But if you have celiac disease and don't know it, you may continue to eat a diet containing gluten. That gluten keeps working away at the intestines, and the symptoms may not go away.

Symptoms of Celiac Disease

Sometimes, people have celiac disease but don't experience gastrointestinal symptoms. In the past, doctors didn't know this was possible, and people could be sick with celiac disease their whole lives and never realize it. We now know that many people with celiac disease have symptoms in parts of the body other than the intestines; they may have no or only mild gastrointestinal symptoms. These atypical symptoms are often caused by the lack of one or more nutrients due to the malabsorption of food resulting from damage to the small intestine. A third group of people with celiac disease may show no symptoms of the disease at all, or only such mild symptoms that they don't realize they're sick. Doctors sometimes refer to these cases as "silent" celiac disease. When one considers the many possible sets of symptoms (or even no symptoms) associated with the condition, plus the fact that most of these symptoms could also be due to other more common ailments, it's no wonder that some individuals may have celiac disease for years before it's finally diagnosed.

In the past, celiac disease was thought to occur only in childhood. Babies afflicted with it typically have diarrhea, often accompanied by slow growth and a swollen belly. These symptoms occur shortly after gluten is introduced into the baby's diet. Many doctors were taught that celiac disease was rare, so they don't think to test for it. Even the classic case of infant celiac disease can go unrecognized for months, and perhaps through visits to several doctors. The diagnostic process may be more lengthy when symptoms first occur in adolescence or adulthood, or if symptoms occur somewhere other than the gastrointestinal tract. Once a patient is suspected of having celiac disease, she will usually be referred to a gastroenterologist for diagnosis and

FAQ

Ten Great Questions to Ask If You Think You Have Celiac Disease

1. Sometimes, I get sick to my stomach and have diarrhea. Could I have celiac disease?

2. A friend in my class has celiac disease. Could I catch it if we share a can of soda?

3. My little brother has celiac disease. Do you think I have it, too?

4. How do you find out if you have celiac disease?

5. My friend has celiac disease, and I'm afraid to invite him to my house. What if he eats something and gets sick?

6. What causes people to get celiac disease?

7. Will it hurt if I eat just a little bit of gluten?

8 Is there a cure for celiac disease?

9 Does it hurt to get tested for celiac disease?

10 I took a chance and went off my gluten-free diet. I feel fine. Does that mean my celiac disease went away?

follow-up care. A gastroenterologist is a physician who specializes in diseases of the gastrointestinal tract.

Scientists do not completely understand why some people with celiac disease have one set of symptoms and others have a different set of symptoms. It may be that gluten affects certain areas of the small intestine in some people, and different areas of the intestine in other people. In particular cases, the symptoms start gradually. In others, the symptoms come on suddenly and severely. There are also instances where symptoms completely go away, only to return in a few weeks or months.

The most commonly recognized symptom, diarrhea, results from several aspects of gluten's damage to the intestines. When the cells of the villi are damaged, fluids can leak into the intestinal tract. Also, when nutrients fail to be absorbed, they pass into the colon. There, they cause the colon to add water to the fecal matter, versus carrying out its normal function of removing water. This excess liquid leads to looser and more frequent bowel movements. Nutrients in the colon can also encourage bacterial growth, contributing excess gas. The additional liquid and gas in the intestines may cause pain, cramps, and bloating.

Other common symptoms of celiac disease result from poor absorption of nutrients, including essential vitamins and minerals. Many cases of the disease are first suspected when a symptom indicates a shortage of one of these essential nutrients. However, as with gastrointestinal symptoms, symptoms due to poor absorption are associated with many other diseases as well. Reduced absorption of the major nutrients (carbohydrates, protein, and fats) leads to weight loss, slow body growth, and fatigue. If damage to the small intestine prevents the absorption of sufficient iron, a person may develop a form of anemia, in which there is a shortage of red blood cells to carry oxygen throughout the body. Failure to absorb sufficient calcium can affect bone growth, as well as cause symptoms such as back and leg pain, and muscle twitching. There are many other vitamins and minerals that the body requires in small amounts, and a shortage of any of these can lead to a wide variety of ailments.

Testing for Celiac Disease

If you think you have celiac disease, consult a doctor about getting tested for it. The tests measure the effects of gluten in the body, so you should visit the doctor while still eating foods with gluten. Otherwise, you will not get accurate results. There are three

The first step in determining if a person has celiac disease is to test a blood sample for evidence of celiac-associated antibodies.

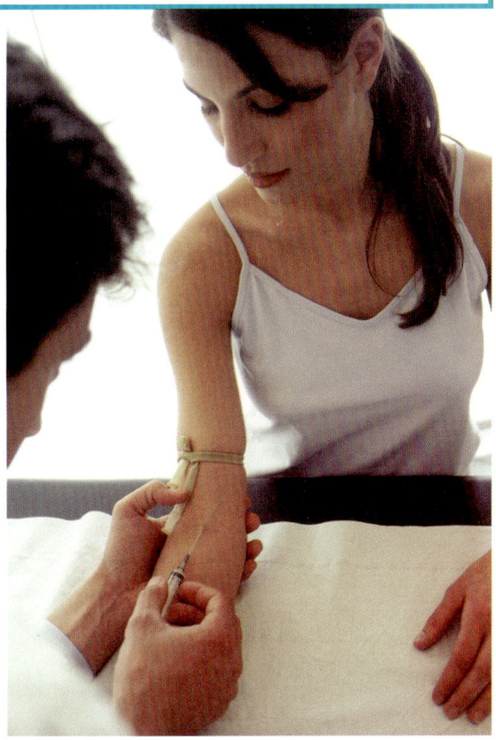

phases to testing for celiac disease. Your gastroenterologist will administer the first test, then wait for the results. Once he knows the results, he will determine if the second and third phases are necessary.

The first phase in the diagnostic process involves testing for certain chemicals in a sample of blood. Only a small sample is taken, and this is usually done in a doctor's office or laboratory. Several blood tests are available, but the best ones, as recommended by a panel of experts convened by the U.S. National Institutes of Health, test for tissue transglutaminase (TTG) and endomysial antibodies (EMA). TTG is the enzyme that makes gluten toxic to a person with celiac disease, as we learned in chapter 1. If the blood contains an antibody to TTG, it means the person probably has celiac disease. Both of the tests are highly reliable, but not 100-percent reliable. In a few cases, a person with celiac disease may test negative on one

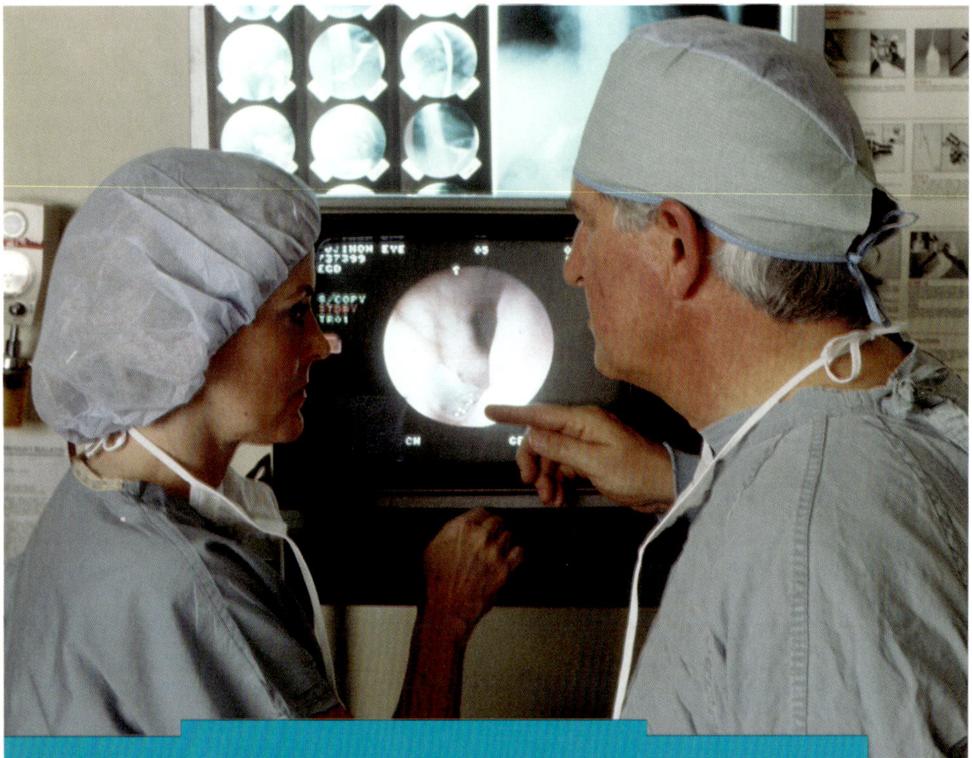

These doctors are examining pictures from an endoscopy procedure. This procedure allows doctors to see if there is damage to the lining of the small intestine. It is the most important test for celiac disease.

or both tests. Other diseases, like diabetes, may cause a positive TTG test. Also, the tests are not ideal for diagnosing very young children.

In the second phase of testing, called endoscopy, the gastroenterologist actually looks at the inside of the small intestine. He is looking for evidence of damage caused by exposure to gluten. The procedure is done at a hospital. It takes only a short while and usually doesn't require staying overnight. The person is sedated or given general anesthesia (put to sleep) prior to the procedure. She does not feel anything or remember anything once it is over. A small tube is inserted through the mouth and threaded through the stomach to the duodenum portion of the small intestine. The doctor is then able to look through the tube to examine the lining of the intestine and to take a small tissue sample (biopsy). A doctor will later examine the tissue under a microscope. He will be looking for any flattening of the villi on the intestinal lining. If the villi are damaged, this means that the body has been reacting to gluten, and the test is positive for celiac disease.

If someone has both a blood test and intestinal biopsy that are positive for celiac disease, the gastroenterologist will then recommend the third part of the test. This consists of eating a diet that totally excludes foods containing gluten. If symptoms go away in a few weeks or months, it is certain that the individual has celiac disease. Every case of the disease is different, and doctors may sometimes recommend different tests for some people. However, experts regard the three phases of testing described above as the most certain way to diagnose celiac disease. It is very important to be sure one has the disease before making a lifelong change in eating.

Dermatitis Herpetiformis

You may hear of someone who does not eat gluten because he has a skin disease. He has another form of celiac disease, called dermatitis herpetiformis. About 10 percent of people with celiac

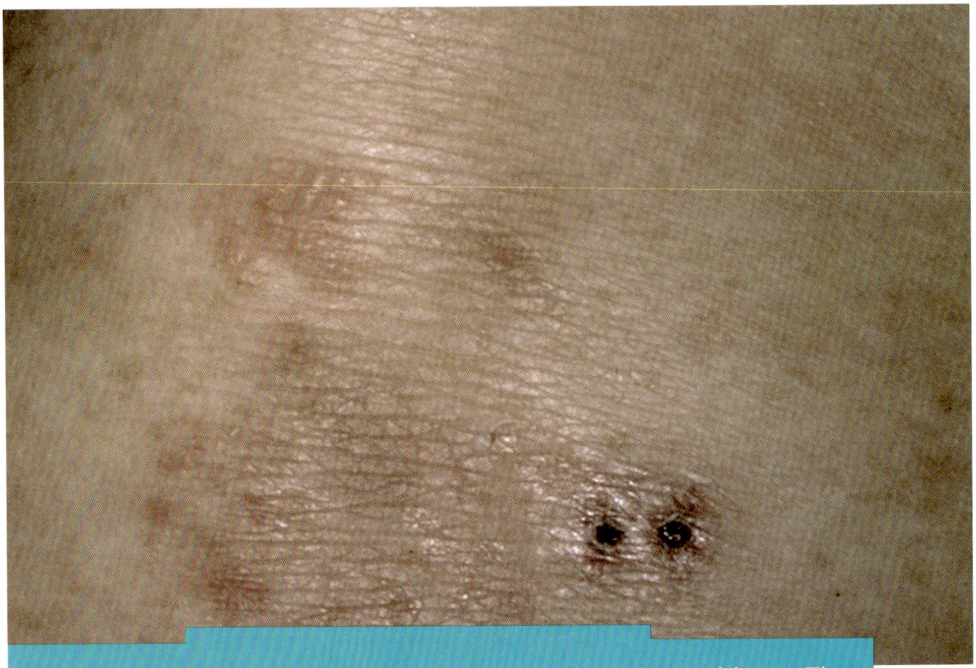

One form of celiac disease causes a skin rash, pictured here. The rash is extremely itchy. Persons with this form of the disease may or may not have intestinal symptoms.

disease have this form of the disease. It rarely occurs in children. The chief symptom is an extremely itchy skin rash with blisters. The rash is caused by an immune reaction to gluten. The intestines may or may not be affected in this form of the disease, but the treatment is the same—a gluten-free diet. Dermatitis herpetiformis is diagnosed by a biopsy examination of a small sample of skin.

Chapter three

WHO GETS CELIAC DISEASE?

When ancient people lived as nomads and hunted for food, there was no grain like our modern-day wheat in their diet. Over thousands of years, humankind evolved and began to domesticate animals and food crops. New foods such as milk and cultivated grains became dietary staples. Yet digestive systems were not always adapted to process these foods. We know from early history that various digestive complaints were commonplace. One disease record from second-century AD sounds much like what we know today as celiac disease.

Discovering the Link to Gluten

Parents become worried when a young child has intestinal symptoms and fails to grow properly. In the past, doctors

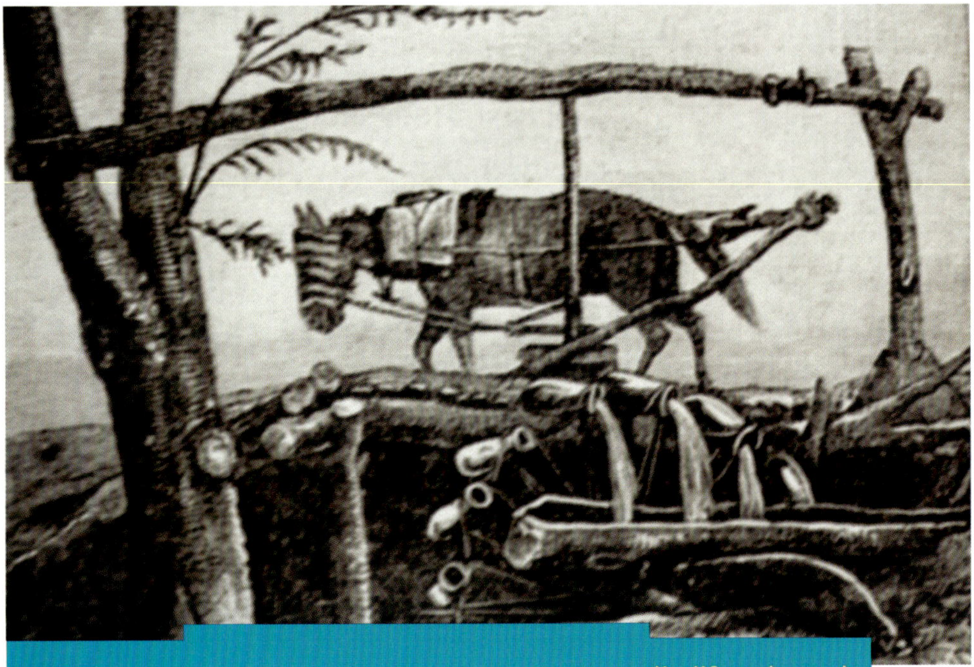

In ancient times, our ancestors gave up a nomadic lifestyle and began to cultivate crops, such as wheat. This photo shows an early crop irrigation system.

treated these children as best they could, but often nothing helped. It was not until the 1940s that the link between celiac disease symptoms and eating gluten was first noted. This came about when the Netherlands was occupied by the German army during World War II. Food was scarce, and the native Dutch were forced to survive mainly on potatoes and rice. Dr. Willem Karel Dicke was a Dutch pediatrician, and he had been treating several children who had severe intestinal problems. When the food scarcity caused by the war forced these children to survive on a diet without wheat, Dr. Dicke

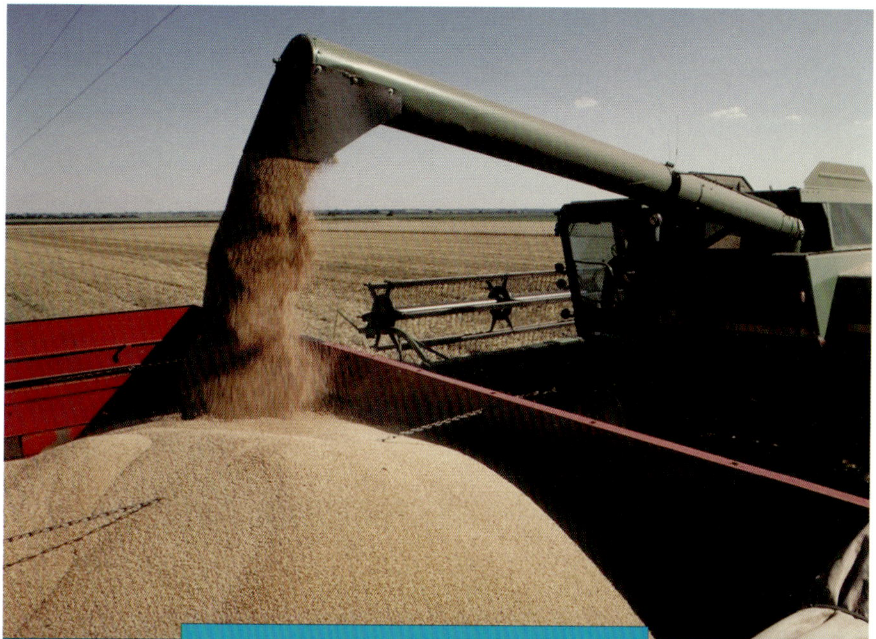

Wheat grows abundantly in moderate climates throughout the world. Foods based on wheat have become staples in many cultures.

noted that these children felt better. After the war, when wheat was again available and the children's symptoms returned, Dr. Dicke correctly identified wheat as the cause of their intestinal distress.

Since the 1950s, doctors have understood that removing gluten (the troublesome ingredient in wheat) from the diet is the only required treatment for celiac disease. Still, it has been a slow process for doctors to recognize the symptoms of celiac disease in their patients. For many years, medical professionals in Europe tended to be more aware of the condition and diagnosed it more frequently than those in the United States. For a time, it was thought that celiac disease was more common in Europe than elsewhere. Recent studies show this is not the case. Celiac disease is fairly common in Europe, North America, Asia, Africa, and Latin America. As improved means of testing have been discovered, doctors are now able to diagnose it even when it occurs in its silent form.

Higher Risk Groups for Celiac Disease

As we learned in chapter 1, genetic abnormalities linked to celiac disease occur in many people. Not all of these people develop the disease. Scientists have still not discovered the trigger mechanism that activates the autoimmune reaction to gluten in some people. It's more common among girls: approximately 3 out of 4 people with celiac disease are female. Because it is a genetic disease, it tends to run in families. People who have a close relative (parent, sibling, child) with celiac disease are more likely to have it. When someone tests positive for it, a health professional will likely recommend that close relatives be tested as well.

Persons who have one autoimmune disease are more likely to develop another one. It may be that some genetic abnormality leads to more than one of these diseases. Type I diabetes is an autoimmune disease in which the immune system attacks cells of the pancreas. It occurs most commonly in children. Recent research has shown that as many as 10 percent of children with Type I diabetes will develop celiac disease. Certain

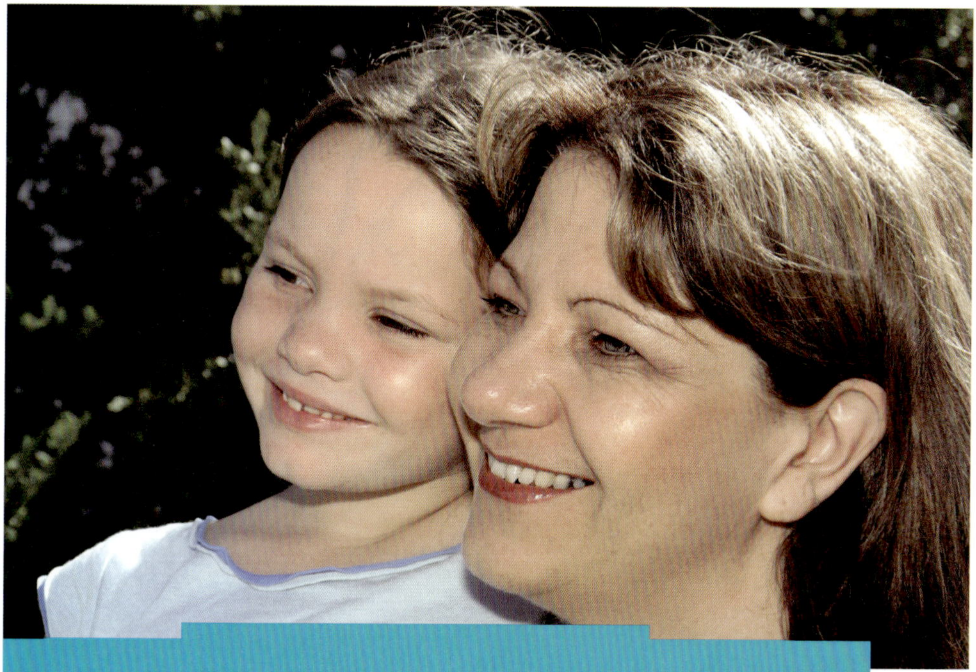

Celiac disease is genetic and may occur in more than one family member. It is more common among girls than boys.

other diseases such as peripheral neuropathy, Down syndrome, and thyroid disease are sometimes associated with celiac disease. If a person has one of these diseases and has gastrointestinal symptoms, testing for celiac disease may be advised.

chapter four

HOW WILL CELIAC DISEASE AFFECT MY LIFESTYLE?

Persons with celiac disease have a serious, lifelong illness that they must deal with every day. On the other hand, they have a condition that is totally treatable, and they can lead a lifestyle that's normal in every way. They must pay attention to what they eat—but shouldn't everyone do that? The recognition of celiac disease as being fairly common makes it easier to deal with. Many grocery stores now carry a variety of gluten-free products (in addition to the huge selection of foods that have never contained gluten, of course). Plus, more people have friends or family members with the disease.

Just Diagnosed with Celiac Disease?

Perhaps the toughest part of having celiac disease is going through the diagnostic procedures, and then learning to

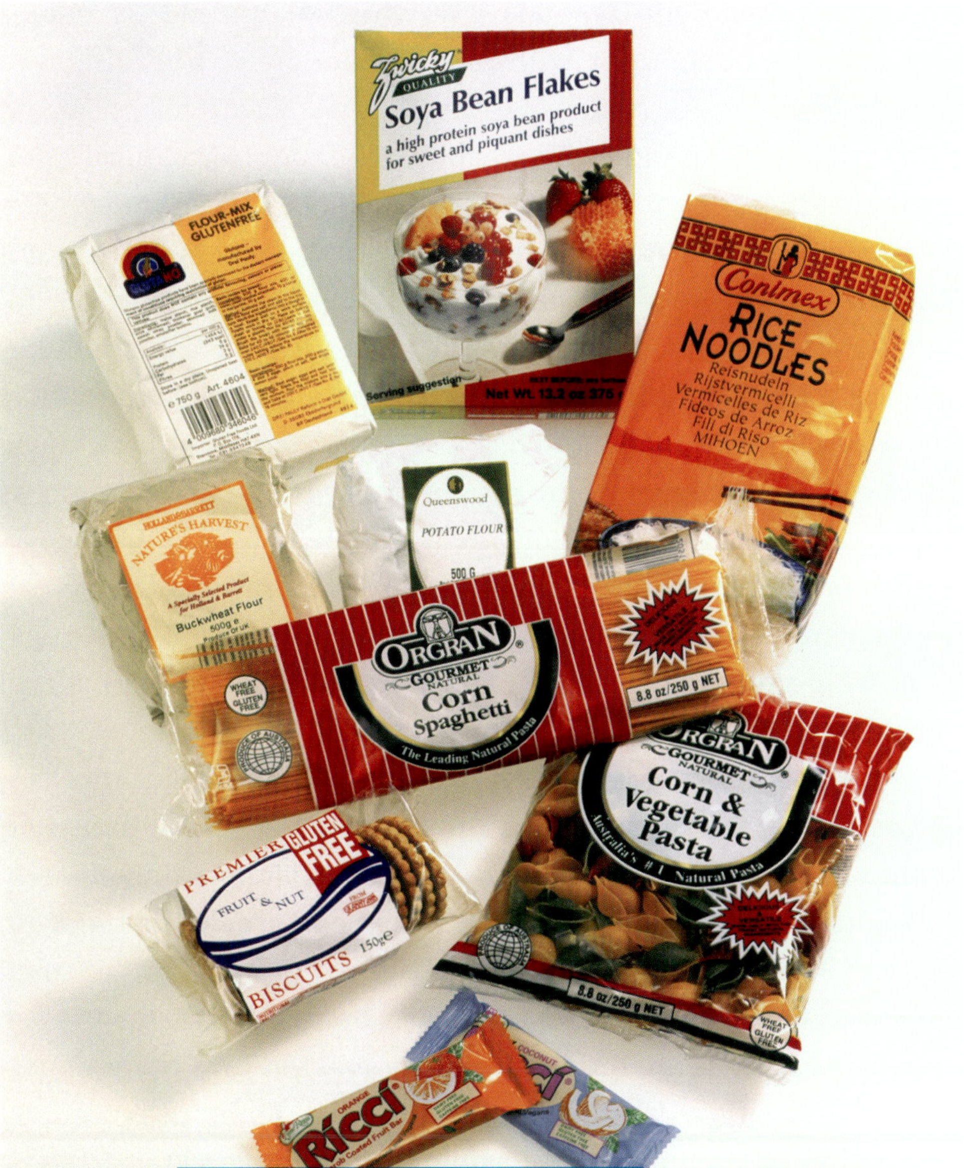

Many gluten-free products are available by mail or from specialty grocery stores. Rice, beans, corn, and nuts are often substituted for wheat.

eat gluten-free. Even persons who were diagnosed as babies may still face challenges with diet management. In addition to dietary changes, a celiac disease diagnosis can bring about many emotional changes. There may be feelings of panic, anger, denial, sadness, or longing to be just like everyone else. The good news is that virtually everyone eventually gets to the point of realizing that how one eats is really just a small part of life. Still, it can seem like a big thing to say no to a luscious-looking piece of a friend's birthday cake when it's all a new experience. If you or someone you know has just been diagnosed with celiac disease, this is a time when support from friends and family is really needed. Plus, the more information you get, the better. Health professionals are your best sources of information, so ask doctors, nurses, technicians, and nutritionists plenty of questions. There are no "one-size-fits-all" answers, so don't be afraid to be specific when you're concerned about something.

What happens after a person is diagnosed with celiac disease? Of course, the first thing to think about is getting back to feeling healthy. For some people, this may happen almost immediately once gluten is removed from their diet. Sometimes, the recovery can take longer, depending on the extent of damage to the small intestine. A doctor may recommend additional medical tests to see if poor absorption of certain foods has created any other conditions that require treatment. Around this time, it is usually recommended that parents and siblings have a blood test to see if they may also have celiac disease. Family members are much more likely to have the disease because of shared genetics. Celiac disease is not contagious, so friends have nothing to worry about.

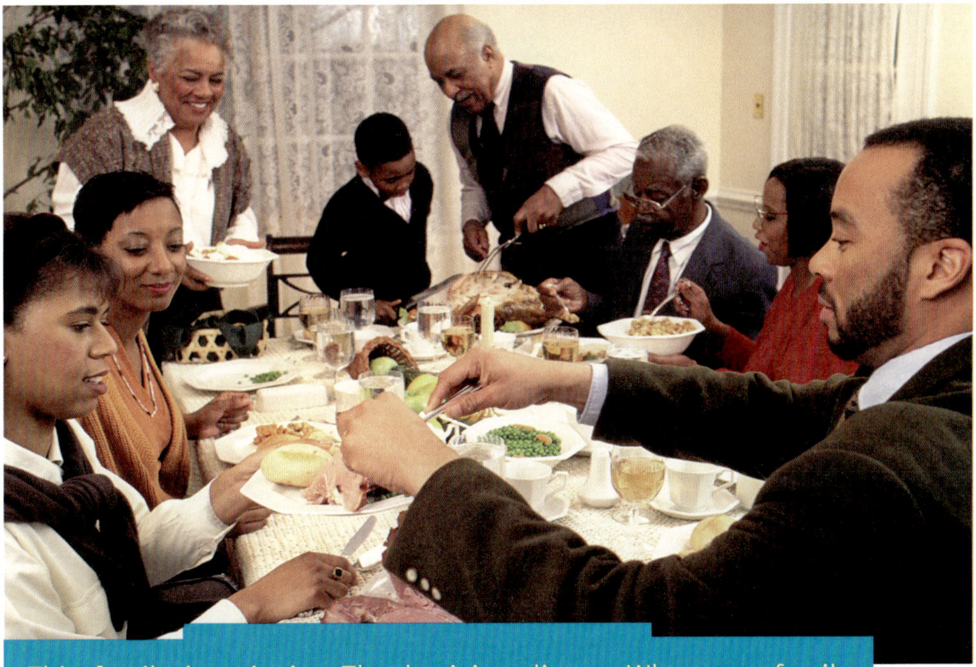

This family is enjoying Thanksgiving dinner. When one family member has celiac disease, the whole family can help him with his gluten-free diet.

Keeping at It, Gluten-Free

As years go by, the temptation to go off a gluten-free diet is just too great. Or one may decide that giving up so many fun foods is not worth it. If a bout of "gluten gluttony" results in no intestinal upset, the individual may decide she doesn't have celiac disease after all, or that she has "outgrown" it. This is why it's so important for the initial diagnosis of celiac disease to be established by medical specialists, as described in chapter 2. If someone truly has the condition, it does not go

BECKY'S STORY

The conductor raises his baton for the downbeat. Becky is on the edge of her chair, watching for his signal. It's exciting to be playing her flute with an orchestra for the very first time. The audience looks huge! Her parents and little brother are out there watching, and she's eager to do her best.

When she's not playing flute, Becky is busy with lots of other activities. She's a good student. She also plays on her school soccer team. Becky likes all kinds of music, enjoys summer camping vacations with her family, and has lots of friends. In short, she's a typical teenager. Oh, and she has celiac disease. To her, it's just a part of living. It means she's careful about what she eats. But what's the big deal about that? Her mother is able to buy gluten-free foods at the grocery store, and she and Becky know how to cook all Becky's favorite foods. Her dad helps out by stocking the freezer with gluten-free pizza crusts from the recipe he's perfected over the years. Becky can pull one out and load it up with toppings when it's her night to cook the family supper or when friends come over. Sometimes, she whips up a big pot of spaghetti and sauce, using gluten-free pasta. Her whole family eats it, since they've decided they like the gluten-free version better.

Becky is the only one with celiac disease. The rest of her family eats bread and other foods containing gluten, but they're careful to keep crumbs away from anything Becky might eat. Sometimes, when Becky goes to her friends' houses, she takes along her own snacks to be sure she has something gluten-free to eat. But most of her friends know she has celiac disease, and they find it an adventure to prepare foods that Becky can eat. They like playing detective and know all about reading food labels to look for gluten that might be hiding away under another name in the marshmallows or pudding mix.

Becky's parents found out she had celiac disease when she was only a year old. They immediately learned all about how to feed Becky a healthy diet that didn't contain gluten. Becky doesn't remember ever eating foods with gluten in them or how sick they made her when she was a baby. Maybe this makes it easier for her to eat right, since she eats the same foods she's always known and enjoyed. A few times, she has been sick to her stomach and her mother thinks Becky may have eaten some gluten without knowing it. After that, she's been very careful and has learned to say "no, thank you" if she's offered food she's not sure about.

Her friend Darla is two years older and also has celiac disease. Their mothers found out about each other through an Internet support group. Since Darla's older, she has more experience with things like going to parties. She tells Becky how to eat gluten-free at parties without any embarrassment. It's nice to have an older friend with celiac disease who can give such useful advice.

And the music begins . . . it sounds great. That huge audience is standing up and applauding!

away, even if the symptoms do. If an individual ever has doubts about whether she still has celiac disease, she should question her doctor.

Even without the accompanying symptoms, celiac disease will continue to wage war in the small intestine of an individual who does not follow a gluten-free diet. Several negative consequences are associated with long-term intestinal damage and the resulting lack of certain nutrients. Deficiencies of some minerals and vitamins can damage the nervous system, which may lead to convulsions, loss of feeling or function in the arms or legs, or pain. Untreated celiac disease is associated with infertility in both males and females, probably due to the lack of absorption of nutrients necessary for the function of sex hormones. Osteoporosis, or a thinning of the bones, can result if not enough calcium or vitamin D is available. Both of these are normally absorbed in the small intestine. The risk of developing cancer is about twice as great among celiac patients as in the general population. Cancer of the small intestine, in particular, is more likely among those with celiac disease. Fortunately, the higher risk of cancer generally goes away after a person has been on a gluten-free diet for five years.

We all count on help from family and health professionals, but in the end, we're responsible for making our own healthy eating choices. Lots of people have dietary restrictions due to being overweight or underweight, food allergies, or personal beliefs. A gluten-free diet is one of many, though perhaps with more serious consequences. Once a gluten-free lifestyle is established, most people with celiac disease can move on to other things and

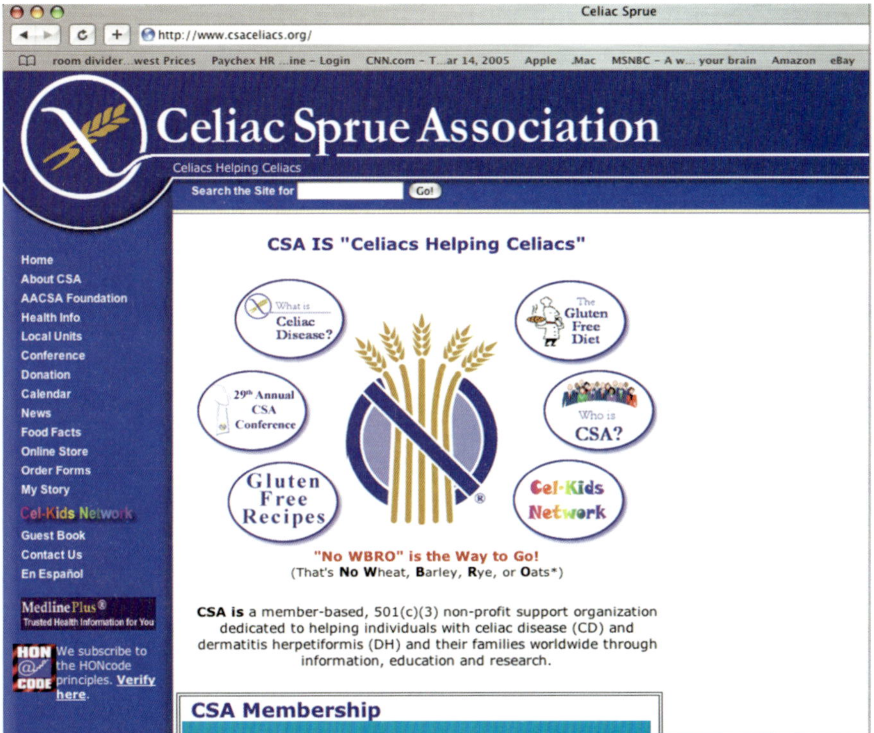

If you have celiac disease, there are organizations ready to provide you with information and support. They can most easily be contacted through the Internet.

realize that eating is not the center of life. And there are still lots of delicious things to eat that don't contain gluten!

Finding Others Who Know What It's Like

Many people with celiac disease find it helpful to join a support group. These groups can provide lots of practical information about where to obtain gluten-free foods, gluten-free recipes, and how to manage eating at restaurants and when traveling. They also can provide the type of support that can only come from someone else who's "been there." Some groups organize summer camps where you can eat everything in sight, since the entire camp is gluten-free. Contact information for groups specializing in celiac disease is listed in the For More Information section of this book. The Internet is also a valuable source of health and food information. However, as with all information on the Internet, be scrutinizing.

chapter five

HOW DO I EAT GLUTEN-FREE?

OK, you're hungry for a hamburger with all the trimmings. No problem. You just order one without the bun and you're gluten-free, right? Wrong! This may work at your favorite neighborhood burger spot where you've previously chatted with the cook. But in a new place, there are questions to be asked. What if the burger isn't made of pure beef, but is hiding a wheat-based filler? Maybe it's cooked on the same grill where buns are warmed. And those French fries were probably cooked in oil that contains bits of breaded onion rings from a previous order.

When you first start a gluten-free diet, it can seem like the whole world is conspiring to hide gluten in everyday food. The first thing you learn is the obvious: no wheat, no rye, no barley. That seems pretty straightforward. The next thing you learn is that some form of these products may be found in a huge variety of

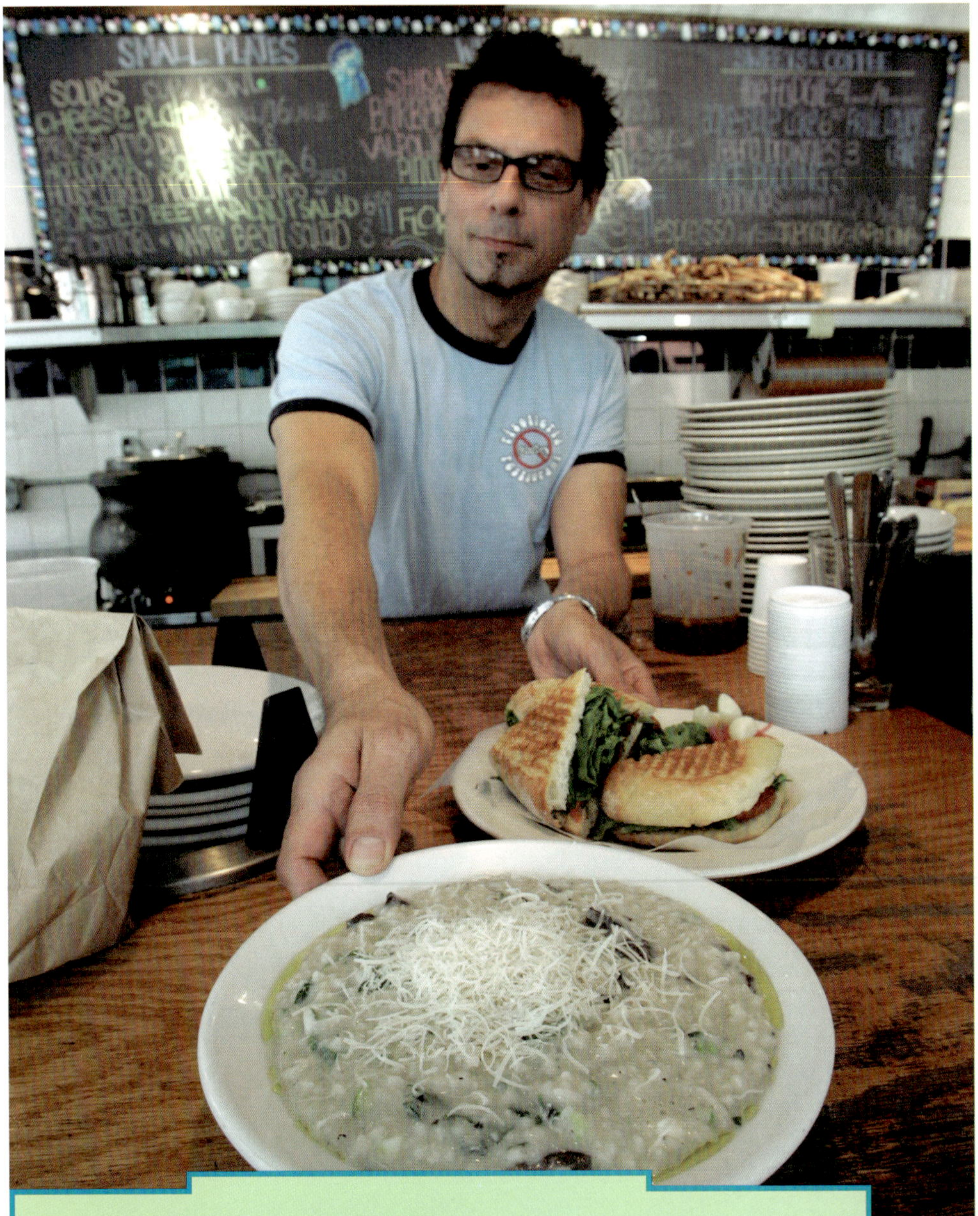

Joe Pace, the owner of Risotteria Restaurant in New York City, serves up gluten-free dishes. His restaurant caters to persons with celiac disease.

foods, and they go by zillions of different names. It can take some time to get the hang of gluten-free eating. Fortunately, it becomes a bit easier these days as more cooks and food servers become familiar with celiac disease. Also, many cookbooks featuring gluten-free recipes are available, and more grocery stores carry gluten-free products. What follows is a brief guide to help you think about what's involved in maintaining a gluten-free diet.

A Variety of Gluten-Free Options

A person with celiac disease has the same need for a nutritious, balanced diet as everyone else. In addition to lots of fruits and vegetables, nutritionists recommend that everyone eat six to eleven servings of bread and cereal every day. Gluten-free products made from rice flour, like bread and pasta, are the most readily available in this food group. Lots of other non-wheat flour sources are those made from corn, potato, flaxseed, beans, and nuts. Several brands of gluten-free breakfast cereal can be found at the grocery store. Just about any favorite recipe can be adapted to the use of gluten-free products. With a bit of planning, a well-balanced diet of everyday foods can be gluten-free. It also provides a chance to sample a wide variety of tasty foods, including many delicious ethnic dishes.

Contamination of Food and Utensils

Unintentional contamination of food is a constant hazard when you're trying to be gluten-free. If you've been eating this way for

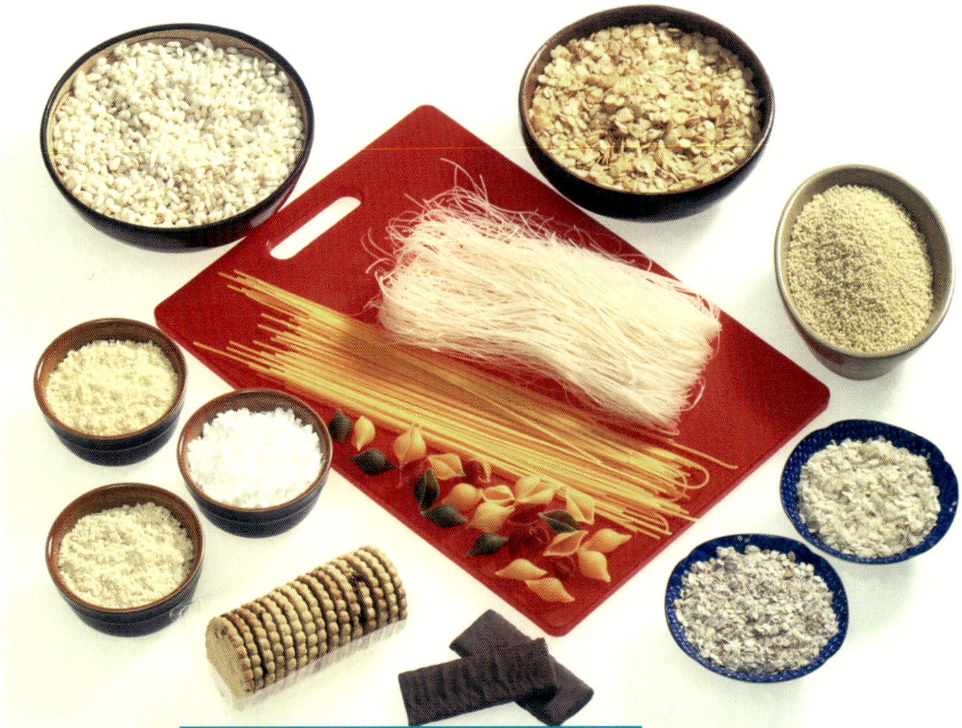

Here is a wide selection of gluten-free foods. On the chopping board are rice noodles, corn spaghetti, and corn and vegetable pasta. Clockwise from upper right are soya bean flakes, millet seeds, brown rice flakes, buckwheat flakes, fruit and carob cookies, plain crackers, soya flour, potato flour, corn meal, and rice cereal.

a while, you already know the things to watch out for. These issues are easier to deal with at home, where you and your family are on guard for gluten. You're all in the habit of carefully washing cutting boards, utensils, and countertops. Perhaps you keep two sets of items such as toasters. You use only clean utensils to dip into the butter dish or peanut butter jar. Away from home, if you eat from a buffet, there is the possibility that someone has contaminated a "good" food by using the serving spoon of a nearby "wheat" food. Or a shopper may have carelessly contaminated the bulk bins at the grocery store. The issue of contamination requires constant judgment calls, while recognizing there's a limit to how careful one can be.

Becoming a Gluten Detective

After dealing with the basics of gluten-free bread, crackers, pasta, and cereal, you must go a step further and look for hidden gluten in processed foods. If it were only as easy as looking for the word "gluten"! Food labels rarely mention the component. So, it's up to you to know that common food additives, like hydrolyzed vegetable protein and dextrin, may contain gluten. Lists of foods and food additives that contain gluten are readily available, and should be kept handy if you're eating or cooking gluten-free. (Books and pocket guides may be ordered from celiac disease support groups listed on pages 57 and 58.) It is sometimes necessary to check with a food manufacturer to be sure about a particular product. As a general rule, unprocessed foods such as meats, fish, fruits, vegetables, rice, allowable grains such as quinoa, and beans are the healthiest choices. One can be sure these foods do not contain gluten. Some common foods, like hot dogs and marshmallows, may contain wheat-based ingredients. In most cases, however, a gluten-free brand can be found by careful label reading. Staples such as mayonnaise, ketchup, and salad dressing are readily available in

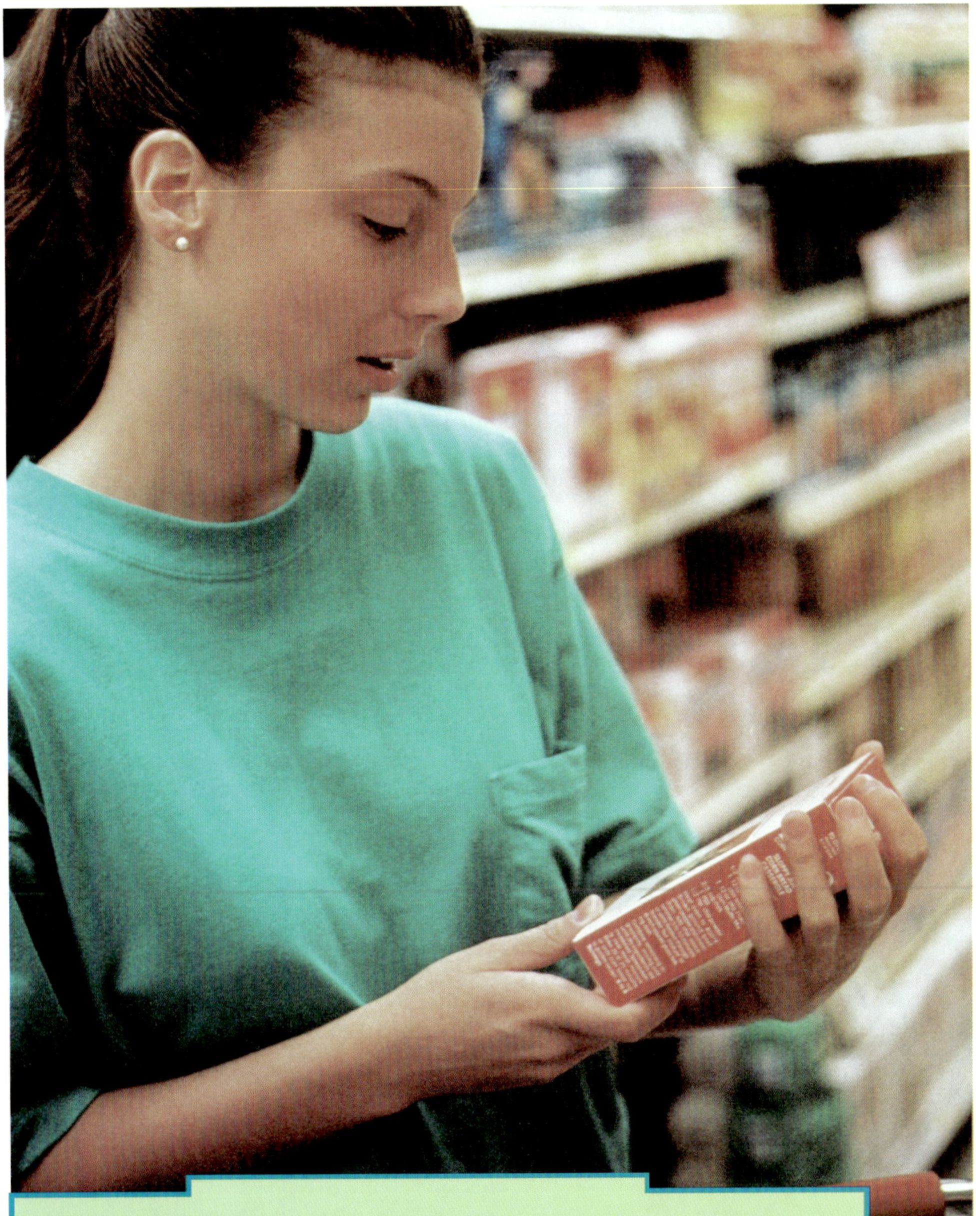

Persons with celiac disease are experts at reading food labels to look for hidden sources of gluten. Beginning in 2008, food sold in the U.S. may be labeled as gluten-free, making food choices easier.

gluten-free form, but the list of ingredients should be checked for forbidden additives. If your favorite brand of a product advertises "New" or "Improved," this would be an excellent time to review the ingredients label to be sure nothing unsafe has been added.

Beginning in 2008, the U.S. Food Labeling Law will allow food processors to add the phrase "gluten-free" to a label if the food is tested and meets agreed-upon standards. Foods imported into this country will have to meet the same requirements to earn the label. Not all foods that are gluten-free will be marked, so it will still be necessary to play detective at times. Still, the availability of "gluten-free" labeling should be a big help.

Eating Away from Home

After you've become skilled in gluten-free shopping and cooking, the next major hurdle is eating away from home. This is where a flexible attitude and a willingness to ask questions really come in handy. People with celiac disease tend to develop a style that works for them. This varies from person to person, and may also vary depending on the situation. The most direct approach to restaurant eating is to select foods that are basic and unadorned, like broiled chicken with no breading, beef without gravy, and salad with oil and vinegar dressing. Be specific with your questions if you're unsure about a menu item, and don't be afraid to let your server or the cook know why you're asking. Some people find it convenient to carry a card they can show to the server or cook that explains the foods they're not able to eat and why it's

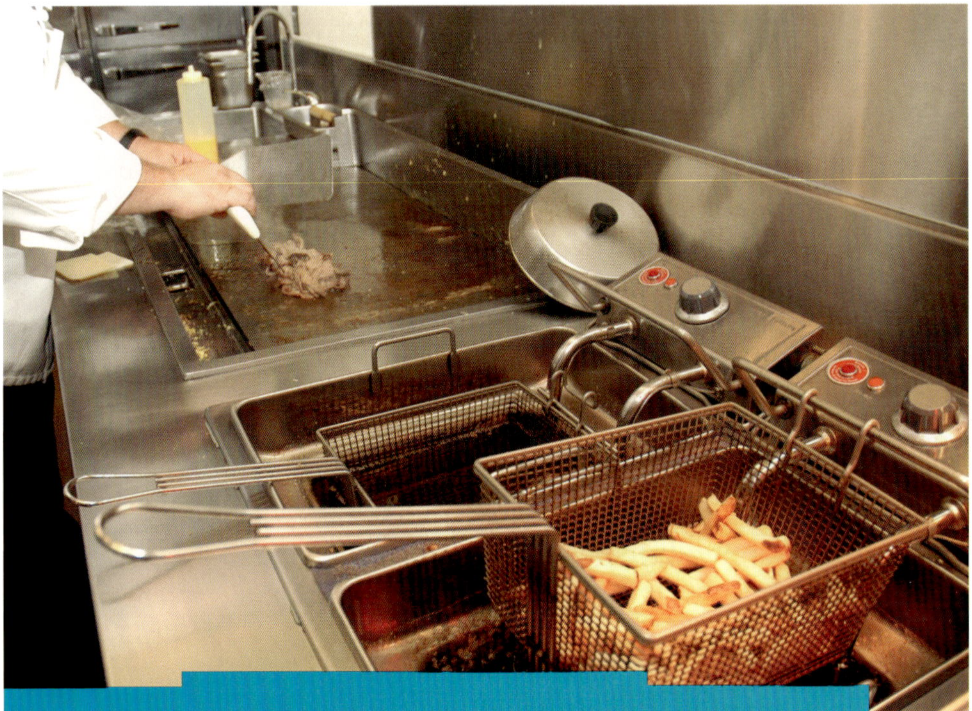

Foods prepared on a fast-food grill may contain bits of gluten. Still, it is possible to order a gluten-free meal when you know the right questions to ask your server.

important. Dessert is probably the most difficult item to order in a restaurant. If you know you'll be somewhere with people ordering dessert, you may want to take along a gluten-free treat you can enjoy along with them. Most restaurants are okay with this when they know the reason. Since traveling may involve eating in many unfamiliar restaurants, you may want to do a little research before you go and have a stash of favorite foods to get you through unexpected situations. Most likely, there will be grocery stores that carry familiar foods you can buy for snacking.

Myths and Facts About Celiac Disease

Myth

Celiac disease is a disease of young children. Fact → Celiac disease may be diagnosed at any age. It may be recognized in babies when they first begin eating foods that contain gluten. However, it is also commonly diagnosed in older children and adults in middle age. Many people experience symptoms of celiac disease for years before they are finally diagnosed.

Myth

Celiac disease is very rare. Fact → Until recently, doctors in the United States regarded celiac disease as being rare and, therefore, seldom tested their patients for it. It is now believed that celiac disease may occur in as many as 1 percent of the U.S. population, or approximately 3 million people.

Myth

The symptoms of celiac disease are intestinal in nature. Fact → Many people are first diagnosed with celiac disease because they have diarrhea, bloating, or weight loss. However, others never experience intestinal symptoms. Instead, they develop an extremely itchy rash, or a condition associated with nutrient deficiency such as anemia. It is also possible to have a "silent" form of the disease and experience no symptoms for many years.

Myth **Celiac disease can disappear after a few years on a gluten-free diet.** Fact → Scientific studies clearly show that once a person shows evidence of an autoimmune response associated with eating gluten, the autoimmune response will never go away. Whenever gluten is eaten, there is the likelihood of further damage to the small intestine and long-term impacts on health. This is true whether or not a person experiences symptoms after eating gluten.

Myth **A little gluten now and then won't hurt anything.** Fact → Scientific studies have not been able to establish limits on amounts of gluten that individuals can eat without damaging their health. Specialists in treating celiac disease uniformly recommend that all persons with the disease adhere as closely as possible to a totally gluten-free diet throughout their lives.

Myth **A person has celiac disease if she feels better after going on a gluten-free diet.** Fact → The diagnosis of celiac disease can only be made for certain after a multiple-step process that involves a biopsy of the intestinal lining, among other things. Because the treatment for the disease requires a lifetime commitment to a strict gluten-free diet, specialists recommend that all individuals who suspect they have celiac disease undergo the complete diagnostic process.

Myth

I must not have celiac disease because my family doctor didn't mention it. Fact → Many doctors are not aware of how common celiac disease is and that it can appear in forms not related to intestinal distress. It has been estimated that the average time required for an individual to be diagnosed with celiac disease may be as long as nine years, after consultation with many doctors.

Myth

Celiac disease is an allergy to wheat. Fact → Celiac disease is an autoimmune disease, meaning that the body mounts an immune response to itself. Gluten (contained in wheat) acts as an initiator of the body's response. Medically, it is a much different process than an allergic reaction. In general, it is a more serious condition because the effects of eating gluten are cumulative and can have long-term consequences.

Myth **People with celiac disease can't wear makeup.**

Fact → Gluten can't be absorbed through the skin, so there is no need for concern about most cosmetic products. Yet some lipstick may contain a wheat-based ingredient. Since a small amount of lipstick may be swallowed, experts advise wearing only those brands known to be gluten-free.

Perhaps the most difficult situations arise when you're invited to someone's home for dinner or out to a special party or event. Of course, if it's your family or a good friend, they already know what foods you like and will probably make a special effort to accommodate you. Your grandmother has probably been baking the holiday turkey separate from the dressing for years. But what about those situations when you'll be among new acquaintances? First off, it's good to remember that lots of people have dietary restrictions of some kind or other, so you're unlikely to be alone in watching what you eat. You may find that your host is busy or you feel uncomfortable asking questions about the food during a party. You could call your host or a caterer before an event to ask about the food being served. Even though you don't want to put your host through extra trouble, it may be very easy for him to do such things as serve gravy on the side rather than with an entrée. This also provides an opportunity for you to offer to bring a gluten-free dish to share, or it may alert you that you should snack beforehand.

What About a Tiny Amount of Gluten Exposure?

If you're eating gluten-free, a common question you may be asked is, "What can it matter to eat one little piece of cake, or even a few bread crumbs?" It is a difficult issue for scientists to study because they don't want to put their patients at risk of too much gluten exposure. So far, they are certain that there can be serious impacts on the body, even if no symptoms are noticeable. Based on currently available evidence, scientists continue to recommend that persons with celiac disease attempt to maintain a totally gluten-free diet. Even tiny amounts of gluten can set off an immune response and result in inflammation of the intestinal lining. Consequences of this process over long periods of time are not completely understood, but scientists think they may be related to the later development of intestinal cancers or additional autoimmune diseases, among other negative effects.

Most people with celiac disease are able to eat oats and oat products without damaging their health. This has been confirmed in clinical studies. Including oats in a gluten-free diet provides additional variety, and is also a healthy source of protein and fiber. Still, some medical professionals don't recommend oats, chiefly because they might be contaminated in the milling and packing process. Individuals keeping a gluten-free diet should rely on their doctors' advice on eating oats.

Lastly, it's good to remember (and reassure your host) that eating a small amount of gluten, either by accident or because you used poor judgment, rarely leads to an emergency situation.

Someone with celiac disease should aim for being gluten-free every single day. The occasional mishap may lead to intestinal upsets that will educate you about something you shouldn't eat and will increase your determination to be even more careful in the future.

Glossary

biopsy Process of taking a small sample of body tissue that is then examined under a microscope to diagnose disease.

coeliac Alternate spelling of celiac, used outside the United States.

crypts Spaces between intestinal villi that secrete fluids into the intestine and regenerate cells of the villi.

dermatitis herpetiformis Form of celiac disease characterized by a blistery skin rash that is extremely itchy.

diabetes mellitus, Type I Autoimmune disease, usually with childhood onset, in which the immune system attacks insulin-producing cells of the pancreas.

diarrhea Liquid stools that occur more frequently than usual bowel movements.

duodenum Upper portion of the small intestine that is important in the absorption of key nutrients. In celiac disease, the reaction to gluten occurs in the duodenum.

endoscopy Medical procedure in which a small tube is inserted through the mouth into the gastrointestinal tract. It allows physicians to observe the intestinal lining and take tissue samples.

gliadin Series of amino acids that make up the portion of the gluten protein that is toxic to persons with celiac disease.

gluten General term that refers to the protein portion of the cereal grains wheat, rye, and barley.

gluten-free diet A diet that excludes gluten in all its forms.

mucosa Lining of the intestinal wall.

neuropathy A condition caused by the inflammation of nerves, resulting in numbness, weakness, or other sensations, often in limbs.

nontropical sprue Alternate name for celiac disease.

osteoporosis Loss of bone density, sometimes leading to fracture.

peristalsis Action of smooth muscles of the intestinal tract with purpose to move food through the digestive system.

sprue Alternate name for celiac disease.

TTG Tissue transglutaminase, an enzyme that acts on gliadin, converting it to a form that is toxic to those with celiac disease.

villi Small projections of tissue in the wall of the small intestine that absorb nutrients from food as it is digested within the intestinal tract.

For More Information

The Celiac Disease Center at Columbia University
630 W. 168th Street, Box 118
New York, NY 10032
Web site: http://www.celiacdiseasecenter.columbia.edu

This is one of North America's largest research and treatment centers for celiac disease. Includes an extensive description of the disease, information on latest research, a section for youth with celiac disease, and an order form for a gluten-free pocket guide and other products.

Celiac Disease Foundation
13251 Ventura Boulevard, Suite 1
Studio City, CA 91604
Web site: http://www.celiac.org

This organization works to increase awareness of celiac disease and provide support for patients, families, and health professionals. Directory of local chapters, including one for young adults. A wide selection of books for sale.

Celiac Sprue Association
P.O. Box 31700
Omaha, NE 68131
Web site: http://www.csaceliacs.org

Support group for persons affected by celiac disease. Web site includes extensive information on eating gluten-free, section for children, health information, and a list of local chapters (including "Cel-Kids Network"). Store section sells a wide variety of publications and products.

National Digestive Diseases Information Clearinghouse
2 Information Way
Bethesda, MD 20892-3570
(A service of the National Institute of Diabetes and Digestive and Kidney Diseases, U.S. National Institutes of Health)
Web site: http://digestive.niddk.nih.gov/
The clearinghouse provides medical information about celiac disease and other digestive disorders, statistics, and links to medical publications.

Web Sites

Due to the changing nature of Internet links, Rosen Publishing has developed an online list of Web sites related to the subject of this book. This site is updated regularly. Please use this link to access the list:

http://www.rosenlinks.com/faq/cedi

For Further Reading

Case, Shelley. *Gluten-Free Diet: A Comprehensive Resource Guide*. 3rd ed. Regina SK, Canada: Case Nutrition Consulting, 2004.

Gluten-Free Living. Magazine, 4 issues per year. Hawthorne, NY. Gluten-Free Living. Back issues and subscriptions available at http://www.glutenfreeliving.com.

Korn, Danna. *Kids with Celiac Disease: A Family Guide to Raising Happy, Healthy, Gluten-Free Children*. Bethesda, MD: Woodbine House, Inc., 2001.

Korn, Danna. *Living Gluten-Free for Dummies*. Hoboken, NJ: Wiley Publishing, Inc., 2006.

London, Melissa, and Eric Glickman. *The GF Kid: A Celiac Disease Survival Guide*. Bethesda, MD: Woodbine House, Inc., 2005.

Reilly, Rebecca. *Gluten-Free Baking*. New York, NY: Simon and Schuster, 2002.

Bibliography

Case, S. "The Gluten-Free Diet: How to Provide Effective Education and Resources." *Gastroenterology* 128S: 128–34, 2005.

Celiac Disease Center at Columbia University. "Diagnosis of Celiac Disease." Retrieved August 30, 2006 (http://www.celiacdiseasecenter.columbia.edu/C_Doctors/C03-Diagnosis.htm).

Fabiani, E., et al. "Compliance with Gluten-Free Diet in Adolescents with Screening-Detected Celiac Disease: A 5-Year Follow-Up Study." *Journal of Pediatrics* 136: 841–3, 2000.

Fasano, A. "Celiac Disease: The Past, the Present, the Future." *Pediatrics* 107: 768–70, 2001.

Fasano, A. "European and North American Populations Should Be Screened for Coeliac Disease." *Gut* 52: 168–9, 2003.

Fasano A. "Celiac Disease—How to Handle a Clinical Chameleon" (editorial). *New England Journal of Medicine* 348: 2,568–70, 2003.

Green, PHR, Jabri, B. *Coeliac Disease*. Seminar. *Lancet* 362: 383–91, 2003.

Green, Peter H.R., and R. Jones. *Celiac Disease: A Hidden Epidemic*. New York, NY: HarperCollins Publishers, 2006.

Lyons, Nancy J. *An Unlikely Foe: Celiac Disease Exposed*. Honolulu, HI: Cotter-Lyons Publications, 2006.

National Institutes of Health Consensus Development Statement. NIH Consensus Development Conference on Celiac Disease. June 28–30, 2004 (http://consensus.nih.gov/2004/2004CeliacDisease).

West, J., et al. "Fracture Risk in People with Celiac Disease: A Population-Based Cohort Study." *Gastroenterology* 125: 429–36, 2003.

Index

G

I

J

M

N

O

P

Q

T

V

About the Author

Terry L. Smith, M.S., is a statistician and science writer living in Lawrence, Kansas. She formerly served on the faculty of the University of Texas M.D. Anderson Cancer Center in Houston, and is a co-author of numerous medical articles. Smith's most recent publication is the book *Breast Cancer: Current and Emerging Trends in Detection and Treatment.*

Photo Credits

Cover © www.istockphoto.com/Jason Stitt; p. 5 © Kwame Zikomo/SuperStock; p. 8 by Tahara Anderson; p. 10 © L. Birmingham/Custom Medical Stock Photo; p. 12 (top) Photo courtesy of USDA Natural Resources Conservation Service; p. 12 (middle and bottom) U.S. Department of Agriculture photos; p. 16 © Adam Gault/Photo Researchers, Inc.; p. 23 © Marka/ Custom Medical Stock Photo; pp. 24, 28 © Custom Medical Stock Photo; p. 26 © Logical Images/Custom Medical Stock Photo; p. 29 Gene Alexander/USDA Photo; p. 31 First Class Photos PTY LTD/Shutterstock.com; pp. 33, 44 © Sheila Terry/ Photo Researchers, Inc.; p. 35 © Chuck Savage/Corbis; p. 39 www.celiacawareness.org; p. 42 © Gregory Bull/AP/Wide World Photos; p. 46 © J. Silver/SuperStock; p. 48 © www. istockphoto.com/Franklin Lugenbeet.

Editor: Leigh Ann Cobb; Series Designer: Evelyn Horovicz
Photo Researcher: Hillary Arnold